# The Easiest Oven Cookbook 2021

Delicious Oven Recipes for Any Day of the Week

# Introduction

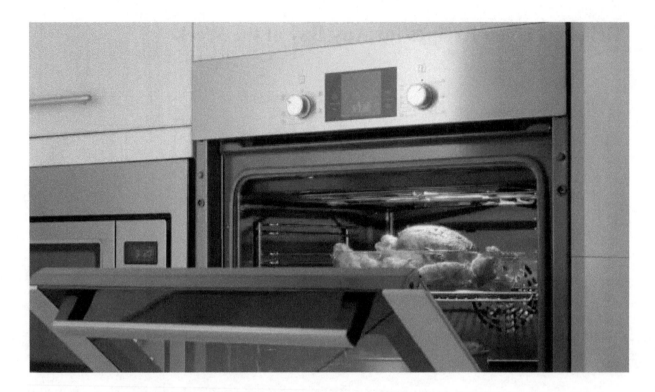

Are you excited to finally be ready to dive in and use that oven of yours? Sure, it can be a very traumatic experience, especially if you have had mishaps in the past resulting in less than juicy meats or darker then expected pastries. Today is the day you say no more! No more will you be afraid of that oven of yours. Ovens are pretty simple to use especially when you know a few best practices to go by. That, my friend is what this Oven Cookbook will help you to get a sense of. By cooking through these 30 simple oven recipes you will learn your way around the oven.

Why not cut all the tension and suspense and just dive right in? Skip the page and let's get started on our first recipe.

## Cheesy Egg Muffins

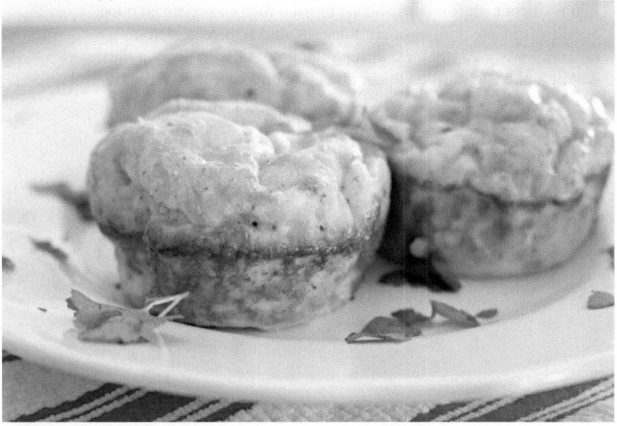

These delicious egg muffins serve as an easy breakfast dish.
**Serves:** 6
**Time:** 30 Minutes
**Ingredients:**

- Eggs (4 large)
- Greek yogurt (2 tbsp., full fat)
- Almond flour (3 tbsp.)
- Baking powder (¼ tsp.)
- Cheddar cheese (1½ cup, shredded)

**Directions:**
1. Preheat oven to 375 degrees Fahrenheit.

2. In a medium bowl, add the yogurt, and the eggs and season with salt and pepper, then whisk to combine.

3. Add your coconut flour and baking powder, then mix to form a smooth batter.

4. Next, add your cheese, and fold to combine. Evenly pour your mixture into 6 silicone muffin cups and set to bake in your preheated oven.

5. Allow to bake until eggs are fully set, and lightly golden on top (approximately 20 minutes, turning the tray at the halfway point).

6. Allow the egg muffins to cool on a cooling rack then serve. Enjoy!

# Cheesy Roasted Brussel Sprouts Salad

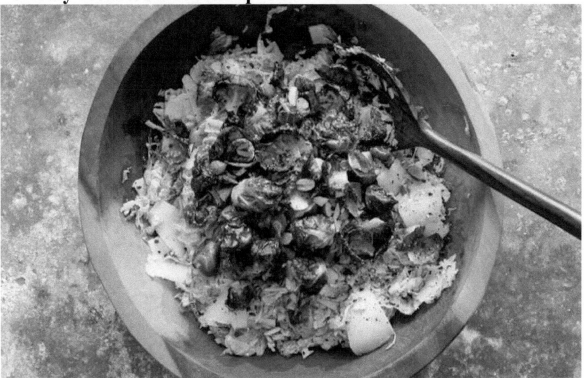

This simple recipe adds a dash of uniqueness to bitter Brussels.
**Serves:** 2
**Time:** 25 Minutes
**Ingredients:**

- Brussels sprouts (1 lb.)
- Olive oil (1 tbsp)
- Feta cheese (1 cup, crumbled)
- Parmesan cheese (¼ cup, grated)
- Hazelnuts (¼ cup, whole, skins removed)
- Pink salt and pepper to taste

1. Preheat your oven to 350 degrees F. Line a baking sheet with a silicone baking mat or parchment paper.
2. Trim the bottom and core from each Brussels sprout with a small knife.
3. Put the leaves in a medium bowl; you can use your hands to fully release all the leaves.
4. Toss the leaves with the olive oil and season with pink salt and pepper.
5. Add your leaves evenly in the bottom of your baking sheet. Roast for 10 to 15 minutes, or until lightly browned and crisp.
6. Divide the roasted Brussels sprouts leaves between two bowls, top each with the shaved Parmesan cheese and hazelnuts, and serve.

# Shredded Brussels Sprouts With Bacon

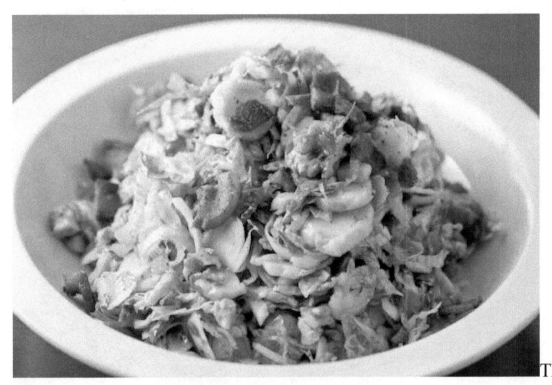

This delicious Brussels dish makes the perfect side to any entrée.

**Serves:** 4
**Time:** 35 Minutes
**Ingredients:**

• Brussels sprouts (6 cups, washed and trimmed)
• Ghee (2 tbsp, melted)
• Garlic (2 cloves, crushed)
• Lemon juice (2 tbsp)
• Bacon (6 pieces, thinly sliced)

1. Preheat your oven to 400 degrees Fahrenheit.
2. Add to your food processor and finely slice using a slicing blade. Mix the ghee with the garlic.
3. Add your sprouts evenly in a large baking sheet, top with a mixture of lemon juice, crushed garlic and melted ghee.
4. Season to taste and add the bacon. Mix until combined.
5. Set to roast for about 20 minutes, stirring a few times during cooking to help it cook evenly. 6. When finished, set to cool slightly then serve.

# Grilled Mediterranean Vegetables

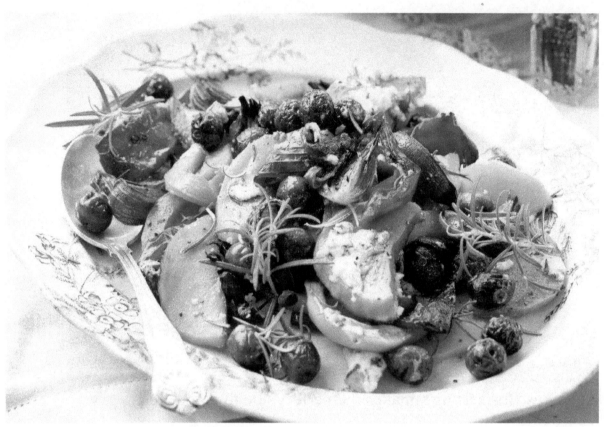

This vegetable dish is delicious and easy to put together.

**Serves:** 6

**Time:** 30 Minutes

**Ingredients:**

• Ghee or butter (1/4 cup)
• Pepper (2 small, red, orange or yellow)
• Zucchini (3 medium, sliced)
• Eggplant (1 medium)
• Red onion (1 medium)
• Salt (3 tsp.)
• Pepper (3tsp.)
• Garlic (2 cloves, crushed)

1. Set your oven on the broil setting on the highest setting then mix your crushed garlic and ghee together in a bowl.
2. Prepare vegetables. Slice bell peppers in haves and deseed. Then, cut bell peppers into thin strips.
3. Slice the zucchini widthwise into 1/4-inch pieces. Wash the eggplant and slice into ¼ in. pieces (roughly ½ cm).

4. Peel and slice the onion into medium wedges and separate the sections using your hands.

5. Place the vegetables in a bowl and add the chopped herbs and ghee with garlic, salt, and black pepper.

6. Transfer your vegetables evenly to your baking sheet or roasting rack.

7. Set to bake for about 15 minutes. Be careful not to burn them. 8. Serve with your favorite savoury dishes.

# Cauli-Pizza Tartlets

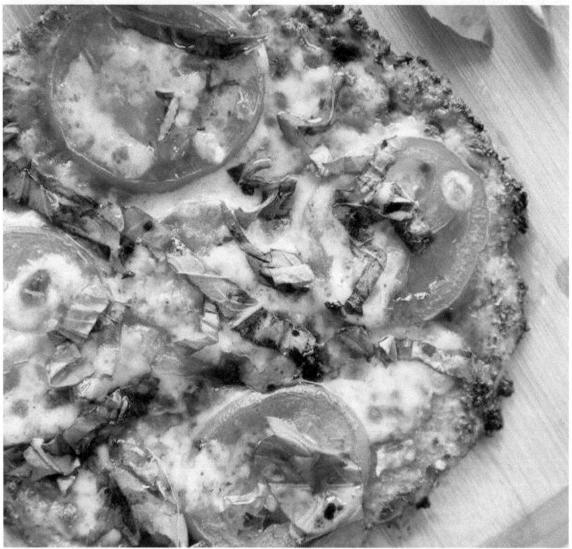

Finally, a healthy version of mini pizzas for your next dinner party appetizer.
**Serves:** 6
**Time:** 30 Minutes
**Ingredients:**

- Rice (2 cups, cooked and dried, cauliflower)
- Cheese (3/4 cup, grated, mozzarella)
- Cheese (1/3 cup, grated, parmesan)
- Egg white (1 large)
- Coconut oil (1 tbsp)
- Salt and pepper to taste

**Directions:**
1. Set your oven to preheat to 400 degrees Fahrenheit.
2. Combine your egg whites, parmesan cheese, half your mozzarella cheese,

and cauliflower rice into a medium bowl, season with salt and pepper to taste then divide evenly into 4 crusts.

3. Brush the crusts with some coconut oil and set to bake until crispy (about 20 minutes).

4. Top with your other half of mozzarella cheese and your favorite toppings. Return to the oven and bake until cheese melts. Enjoy!

# Broccoli Patties

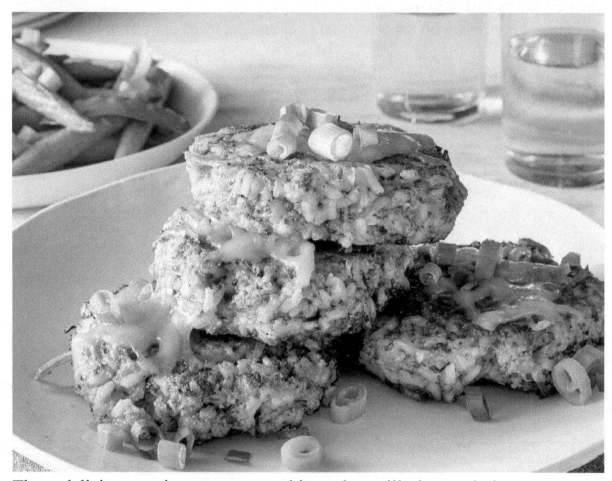

These delicious patties are easy to whip up but will give a whole new reason to love broccoli.

**Serves:** 5
**Time:** 45 Minutes
**Ingredients:**

• Broccoli (1 head, halved florets)
• Lard (2 tbsp)
• Onion (1 medium, white, finely sliced)
• Eggs (3 large)
• Cheese (1/2 cup, grated, cheddar)

1. Preheat the oven to 400 degrees Fahrenheit.
2. Place broccoli on a steaming rack inside a steaming pot filled with approximately 2 inches of water and cook for about 7 minutes.
3. Heat a pan greased with lard and add the onion and crushed garlic. Cook for 5 to 8 minutes until lightly browned.

4. In a bowl, combine your broccoli, pepper, salt and eggs.

5. Add in your garlic and onion then mix until well combined.

6. Using a spoon, create 15 palm-size patties and place them on a baking sheet lined with parchment paper. Transfer to the oven and cook for about 20 minutes or until the tops are lightly browned and crispy.

7. When finished, remove from the oven and set aside to cool or serve immediately.

# Garlic & Herb Cauliflower

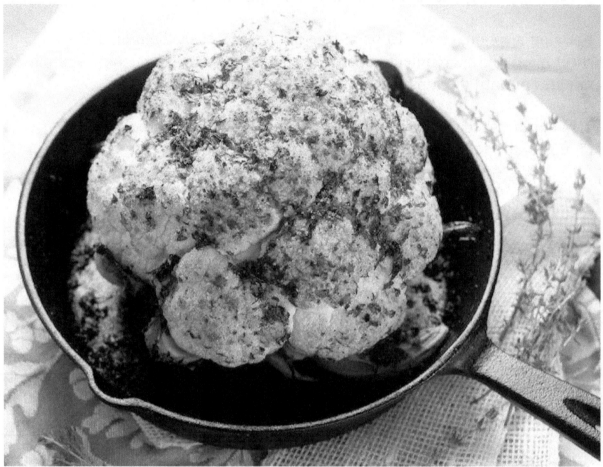

By adding herbs to your roasted cauliflower produces an explosion of flavor.

**Serves:** 4

**Time:** 25 Minutes

**Ingredients:**

- Cauliflower (1 large head, cleaned and cut in florets)
- Butter (1/4 cup, melted)
- Herbs (1/4 cup, chopped, fresh)
- Lemon juice (2 tbsp)
- Garlic (3 cloves, crushed)
- Salt and pepper

1. Preheat the oven to 450 degrees F. Add your cauliflower to a bowl.
2. In another bowl, mix the pepper, salt, garlic, lemon juice, herbs and melted ghee.
3. Add the garlic herb mixture to the bowl with the cauliflower and thoroughly coat. Sprinkle with Parmesan cheese, if using, and place the cauliflower on a baking sheet.
4. Transfer the baking sheet to the oven and bake for 15 minutes or until the

cauliflower turns golden. When finished, remove it from the oven and serve immediately.

# Fish Taco Bowl

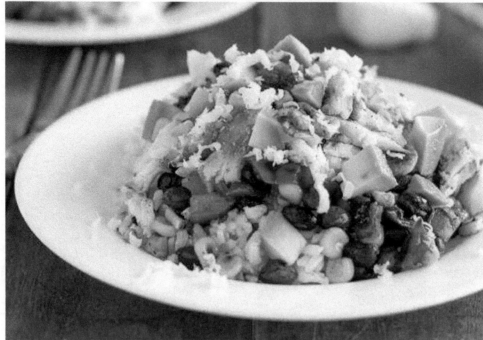

Enjoy all the delicious flavors of a fish taco in one amazing bowl.

**Serves:** 2

**Time:** 25 Minutes

**Ingredients:**

- Tilapia fillets (10 oz)
- Seasoning salt (4 tsp, Tajin, divided)
- Cabbage mix (2 cups, pre-sliced, Cole haw)
- Miso Mayo (1 tbsp, spicy red pepper)
- Avocado (1, mashed)
- Olive oil
- Pink salt and peeper to taste

1. Set your oven to preheat to 425 degrees Fahrenheit. Line a baking sheet with aluminum foil or a silicone baking mat.
2. Rub the tilapia with the olive oil, and then coat it with 2 teaspoons of the Tajin seasoning salt. Place the fish in the prepared pan.
3. Bake for 15 minutes, or until the fish is opaque when you pierce it with a fork. Place the fish on a cooling rack and let it sit for 4 minutes.
4. Meanwhile, in a medium bowl, gently mix to combine the coleslaw and the mayo sauce.
5. Add the mashed avocado and the remaining 2 teaspoons of Tajin seasoning salt to the coleslaw, and season with pink salt and pepper. Divide

the salad between two bowls.

6. Use two forks to shred the fish into small pieces and add it to the bowls. 7. Top the fish with a drizzle of mayo sauce and serve.

# Baked Lemon-Butter Fish

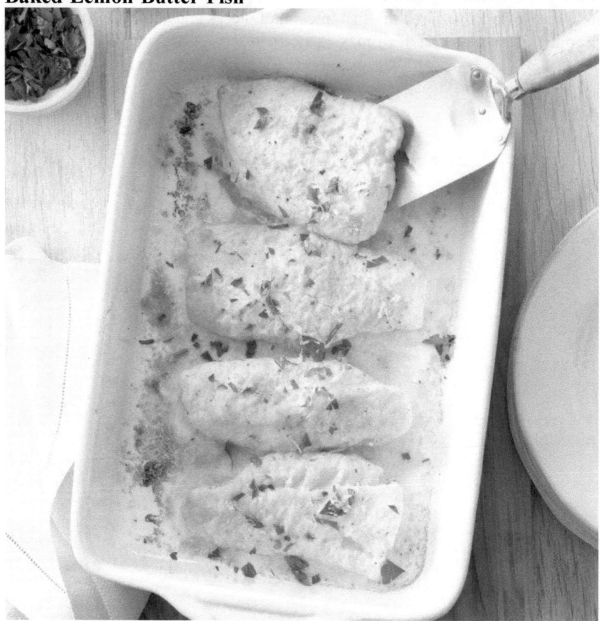

This baked Tilapia is juicy, flaky and delicious.

**Serves:** 2

**Time:** 30 Minutes

**Ingredients:**

- Butter (4 tbsp, plus more for coating)
- Tilapia fillets (2, 5 oz)
- Garlic (2 cloves, minced)
- Lemon (1, zested and juiced)
- Capers (2 tbsp, rinsed and chopped)

**Directions:**

1. Preheat your oven to 400 degrees Fahrenheit and coat an 8-inch baking dish with butter.

2. Pat dry the tilapia fillets with paper towels, and season both sides to taste. Place in the prepared baking dish.

3. Melt the butter over medium heat in a medium skillet. Add the garlic and cook for roughly 3 to 5 minutes, until slightly browned but not burned.

4. Remove the garlic butter from the heat and mix in the lemon zest and 2 tablespoons of lemon juice.

5. Pour the lemon-butter sauce over the fish and sprinkle the capers around the baking pan. 6. Bake for 12 to 15 minutes, until the fish, is just cooked through, and serve.

## Creamy Dill Salmon

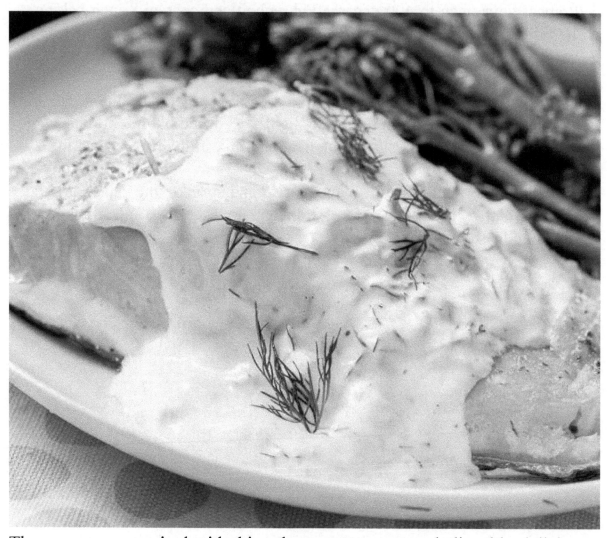

The cream sauce paired with this salmon creates one unbelievably delicious dish.

**Serves:** 2
**Time:** 20 Minutes
**Ingredients:**

- Ghee (2 tbsp, melted)
- Salmon fillets (2 (60z), skin on)
- Mayonnaise (1/4 cup)
- Mustard (1 tbsp, Dijon)
- Dill (2 tbsp, minced, fresh)

1. Preheat your oven to 450 degrees Fahrenheit and lightly grease a baking dish with ghee.
2. Use a paper towel to pat dry the salmon, season to taste with pepper and

pink salt, then place in the baking dish.

3. In a small bowl, mix to combine the mayonnaise, mustard, dill, and garlic powder.

4. Slather the mayonnaise sauce on top of both salmon fillets so that it fully covers the tops.

5. Bake for 7 to 9 minutes, depending on how you like your salmon—7 minutes for mediumrare and 9 minutes for well-done, and serve.

# Parmesan-Garlic Salmon with Asparagus

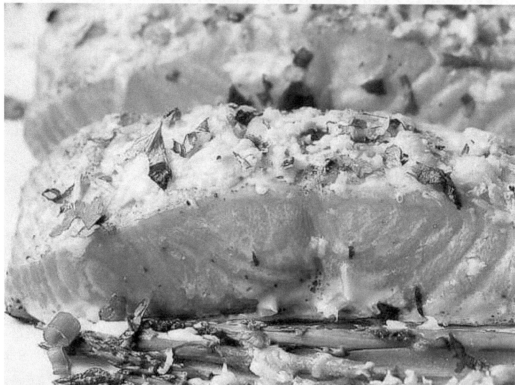

If you like chicken parm then this salmon dish will blow your mind.

**Serves:** 2

**Time:** 25 Minutes

**Ingredients:**

• Salmon fillets (12 oz, skin on)
• Asparagus (1 lb., fresh, trimmed)
• Butter (3 tbsp)
• Garlic (2 cloves, minced)
• Cheese (1/4 cup, grated, parmesan)

1. Set your oven to preheat to 400 degrees Fahrenheit and prepare a baking sheet by lining with foil.
2. Dry your salmon completely, and season to taste.
3. Place the salmon in the middle of the prepared pan and arrange the asparagus around the salmon.
4. Set a skillet over medium heat with butter and allow to melt.
5. Add the minced garlic and stir until garlic begins to brown approximately 3 minutes.
6. Drizzle the garlic-butter sauce over the salmon and asparagus, and top both with the Parmesan cheese.
7. Bake until the salmon is fully cooked, and the asparagus is crisp-tender,

about 12 minutes. Serve.

# Garlic Butter Shrimp

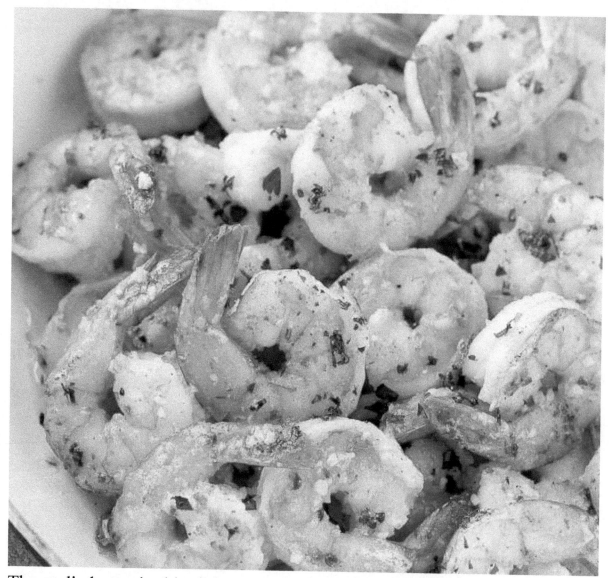

The garlic butter in this shrimp dish add an herby delicious twist to this simple shrimp dish.

**Serves:** 2

**Time:** 25 Minutes

**Ingredients:**

- Butter (3 tbsp)
- Shrimp (1/2 lb)
- Lemon (1, halved)
- Garlic (2 cloves, crushed)
- Red pepper flakes (1/4 tsp)

**Directions:**

1. Set your oven to preheat to 425 degrees Fahrenheit.
2. Place the butter in an 8-inch baking dish and pop it into the oven while it is preheating, just until the butter melts.
3. Sprinkle the shrimp with pink salt and pepper.
4. Slice one half of the lemon into thin slices and cut the other half into 2 wedges.
5. In the baking dish, add the shrimp and garlic to the butter. The shrimp should be in a single layer. Add the lemon slices. Sprinkle the top of the fish with the red pepper flakes.
6. Bake the shrimp for 15 minutes, stirring halfway through.
7. Remove the shrimp from the oven, and squeeze juice from the 2 lemon wedges over the dish. 8. Serve hot.

# Braised Chicken Thighs with Kalamata Olives

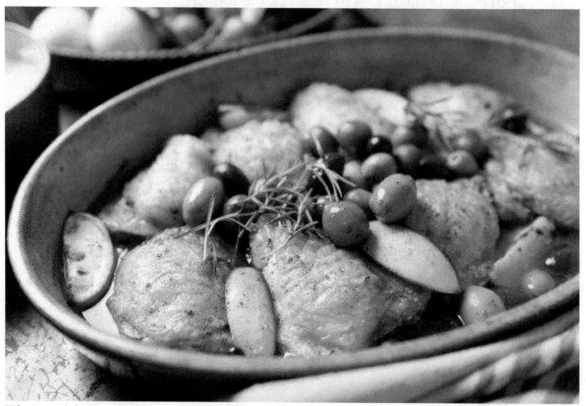

These chicken thighs are complimented by the olives in this braise.
**Serves:** 2
**Time:** 50 Minutes
**Ingredients:**

- chicken thighs (4 pcs, skin on)
- cup chicken broth (1/2 cup)
- lemon (1, ½ sliced and ½ juiced)
- Kalamata olives (1/2 cup)
- 2 tablespoons butter (2 tbsp.)

**Directions:**
1. Set your oven to preheat to 375 degrees F. Dry chicken, and season to taste. 2. In a medium oven-safe skillet, over medium-high heat, melt butter. 3. When the butter has heated and has melted, add the chicken thighs with the skin-side facing the melted butter.
4. Cook until the skin is brown and crispy, roughly 8 minutes.
5. Flip the chicken and cook for 2 minutes on the second side.
6. Around the chicken thighs, pour in the chicken broth, and add the lemon slices, lemon juice, and olives.
7. Bake in the oven for about 30 minutes, until the chicken is cooked through.

8. Add the butter to the broth mixture. 9. Divide the chicken and olives between two plates and serve.

# Parmesan Baked Chicken

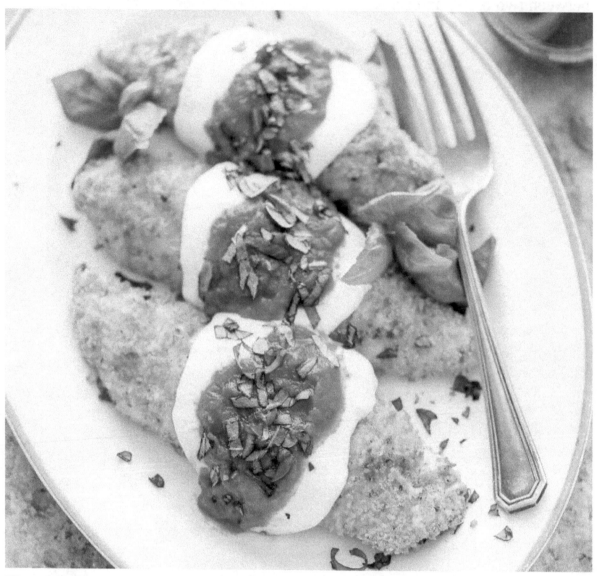

Here is an easy recipe for Chicken parm that will take all your fear away about creating your own chicken parm.

**Serves:** 2
**Time:** 25 Minutes
**Ingredients:**

- ghee (2 tbsp.)
- chicken breasts (2, boneless, skinless)
- mayonnaise (1/2 cup)
- Parmesan cheese (1/4 cup, grated)
- pork rinds (1/4 cup, crushed)
- Italian seasoning (1 tsp.)

**Directions:**

1. Preheat the oven to 425°F. Choose a suitable size baking dish, place both chicken breasts and coat it with the ghee.

2. Pat dry the chicken breasts with a paper towel, season with pink salt and pepper, and place in the prepared baking dish.

3. In a small bowl, combine the mayonnaise, parmesan cheese, and Italian seasoning.

4. Slather the mayonnaise mixture evenly over the chicken breasts and sprinkle the crushed pork rinds on top of the mayonnaise mixture.

5. Bake until the topping is browned, about 20 minutes, and serve.

# Cheesy Bacon and Broccoli Chicken

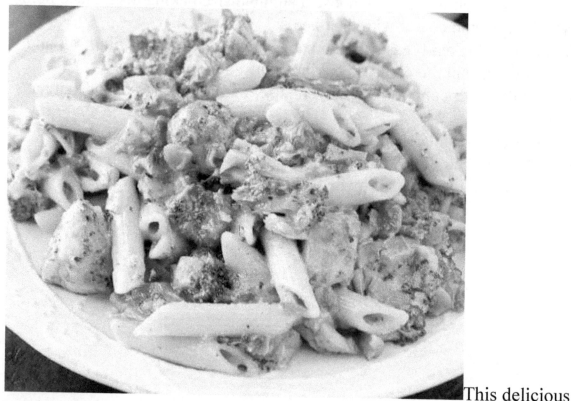

This delicious combo of cheese and broccoli will transform your simple chicken dish into a whole entrée.

**Serves:** 2
**Time:** 1 Hour 10 Minutes
**Ingredients:**

• chicken breasts (2 boneless; skinless)
• bacon (4, slices)
• cream cheese (6 oz., room temp.)
• frozen broccoli florets (2 cups, thawed)
• cheddar cheese (1/2 cup, shredded)
• salt and pepper (to taste)

**Directions:**
1. Set your oven to preheat to 375 degrees F.
2. Choose a baking dish that is large enough to hold both chicken breasts and coat it with the ghee.
3. Pat dry the chicken breasts with a paper towel, and season with pink salt and pepper.
4. Place the chicken breasts and the bacon slices in the baking dish and bake for 25 minutes.
5. Transfer the chicken to a cutting board and use two forks to shred it.

Season it again with pink salt and pepper.

6. Place the bacon on a paper towel–lined plate to crisp up, and then crumble it.

7. In a medium bowl, mix to combine the cream cheese, shredded chicken, broccoli, and half of the bacon crumbles. Transfer the chicken mixture to the baking dish, and top with the Cheddar and the remaining half of the bacon crumbles.

8. Bake until the cheese is bubbling and browned about 35 minutes and serve.

# Buttery Garlic Chicken

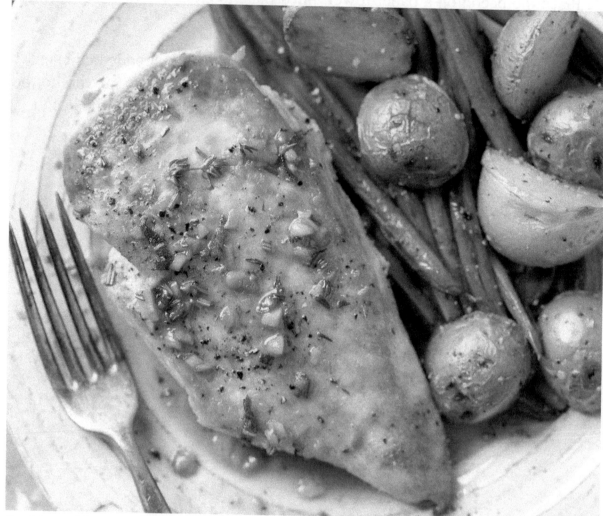

Just as with your shrimp this chicken dish is greatly complimented by this creamy garlicy sauce.

**Serves:** 2

**Time:** 45 Minutes

**Ingredients:**

- ghee (2 tbsp., melted)
- chicken breasts (2 boneless, skinless)
- butter (4 tbsp.)
- garlic (2 cloves, minced)
- Parmesan cheese (1/4 cup, grated)
- salt (1/4 tsp.)
- black pepper (1/4 tsp.)
- Italian seasoning (1 tsp.)

**Directions:**

1. Set your oven to preheat to 375 degrees F. Choose a baking dish that is large enough to hold both chicken breasts and coat it with the ghee.

2. Pat the chicken breasts dry and season with salt, pepper, and Italian seasoning. Place the chicken in the baking dish.

3. Place butter in a medium skillet and melt the butter over medium heat. Add in minced garlic and cook for roughly 4-5 minutes. You want the garlic very lightly browned but not burned.

4. Remove the butter-garlic mixture from the heat and pour it over the chicken breasts.

5. Roast the chicken in the oven for 30 to 35 minutes, until cooked through. Sprinkle some of the Parmesan cheese on top of each chicken breast. Let the chicken rest in the baking dish for
5 minutes.

6. Divide the chicken in two plates, spoon the butter sauce over the chicken, and serve.

# Baked Garlic and Paprika Chicken Legs

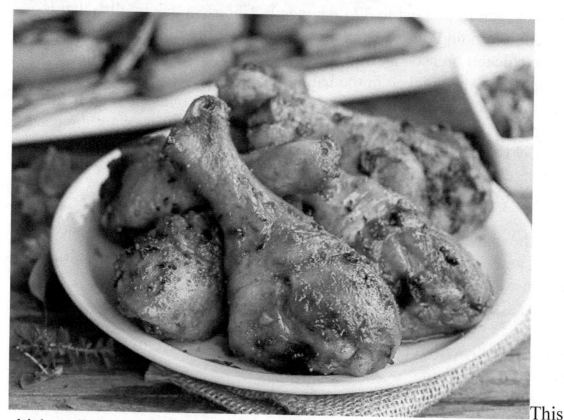

This chicken dish is mildly spicy and savoury.

**Serves:** 2

**Time:** 1 Hour 5 Minutes

**Ingredients:**

- chicken (1 lb., drumstick, skin on)
- paprika (2 tbsp.)
- garlic (2 cloves, minced)
- green beans (1/2 lb., fresh)
- 1 tablespoon olive oil (1 tbsp.)

**Directions:**

1. Set oven to 350°F.
2. Combine all your **Ingredients:** in a large bowl, toss to combine and transfer to a baking dish. 3. Bake for 60 minutes until crisp and thoroughly cooked.

# Parmesan Pork Chops and Roasted Asparagus

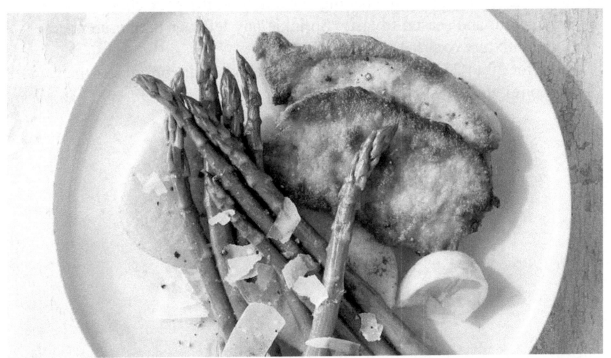

Here we have a simple one pan meal that can be whipped up in a matter of minutes.

**Serves:** 2
**Time:** 35 Minutes
**Ingredients:**

- Parmesan cheese (1/4 cup, grated)
- pork rinds (1/4 cup, crushed)
- pork chops (2, boneless)
- Olive oil, for drizzling
- asparagus spears (½ lb., tough ends snapped off)

**Directions:**

1. Set oven to preheat to 350 degrees F and prepare a baking sheet by lining it with foil.

2. In a medium bowl, combine the Parmesan cheese, pork rinds, and garlic powder and mix well.

3. Use a paper towel to pat the pork chops dry. Season to taste.

4. Place a pork chop in the bowl with the Parmesan –pork rind mixture and press the "breading" to the pork chop, so it sticks. Place the coated pork chop on the prepared baking sheet. Repeat for the second pork chop.

5. Drizzle a small amount of olive oil over each pork chop.
6. Place the asparagus on the baking sheet around the pork chops. Drizzle with olive oil, and season to taste. Sprinkle any leftover Parmesan cheese–pork rind mixture over the asparagus.
7. Bake for 20 to 25 minutes. Thinner pork chops will cook faster than thicker ones. 8. Serve hot.

# Beef and Bell Pepper

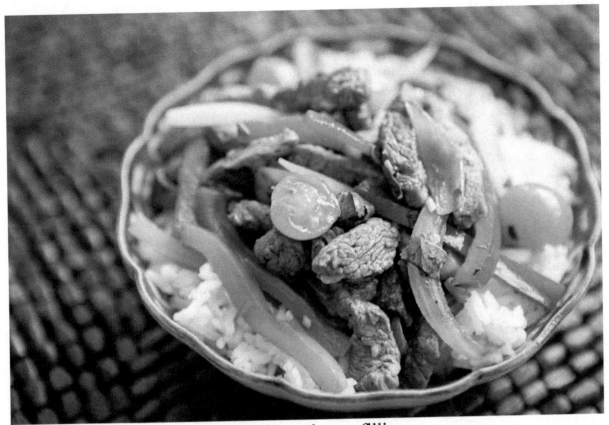

This delicious meal is easy to make and very filling.

**Serves:** 2
**Time:** 30 Minutes
**Ingredients:**

- ground beef (1/2 lb.)
- bell peppers (3 large, in different colors)
- cheese (1/2 cup, shredded)
- avocado (1)
- sour cream (1/4 cup)

1. Set your oven to preheat to 400 degrees F and prepare a baking sheet by lining it with foil.

2. In a large skillet put ghee over medium heat to melt. When the ghee is hot, add beef and season to taste. Stir occasionally with a wooden spoon, breaking up the beef chunks. Continue cooking until the beef is done, 7 to 10 minutes.

3. Meanwhile, cut the bell peppers to get your "potato skins" ready: Cut off the top of each pepper, slice it in half, and pull out the seeds and ribs. If the pepper is large, you can cut it into quarters; use your best judgment, with the goal of a potato skin–size "boat."

4. Place the bell peppers on the prepared baking sheet.
5. Spoon the ground beef into the peppers, sprinkle the cheese on top of each, and bake for 10 minutes.
6. Meanwhile, in a medium bowl, mix the avocado and sour cream to create an avocado crema. Mix until smooth.
7. When the peppers and beef are done baking, divide them between two plates, top each with the avocado crema, and serve.

# Cheesecake Bites Without the Crust

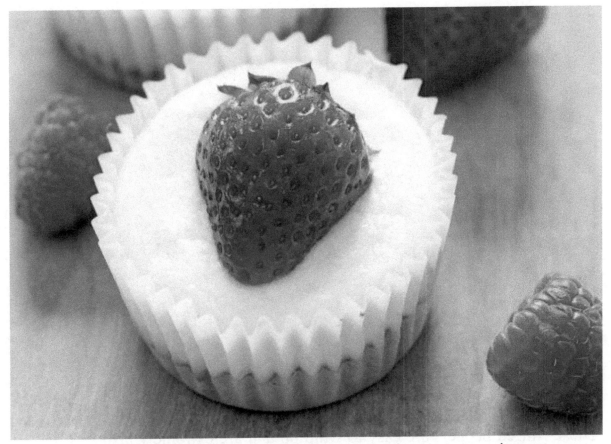

This simple oven made dish is the perfect dessert for anyone trying to cut back on their carb intake.

**Serves:** 4
**Time:** 3 Hours 30 Minutes
**Ingredients:**

- cream cheese (4 oz., at room temperature)
- sour cream (1/4 cup)
- eggs (2 large)
- Swerve natural sweetener (1/2 cup)
- vanilla extract (1/4 tsp.)

1. Preheat the oven to 350°F.
2. Using a hand mixer, into a medium mixing bowl, beat the cream cheese, sour cream, eggs, sweetener, and vanilla until well mixed.
3. Place silicone liners (or cupcake paper liners) in the cups of a muffin tin.
4. Pour the cheesecake batter into the liners and bake for 30 minutes.
5. Refrigerate until well cooled before serving, roughly 3 hours. Store extra cheesecake bites in a zip-top bag in the freezer for up to 3 months.

# Chicken Stuffed Peppers

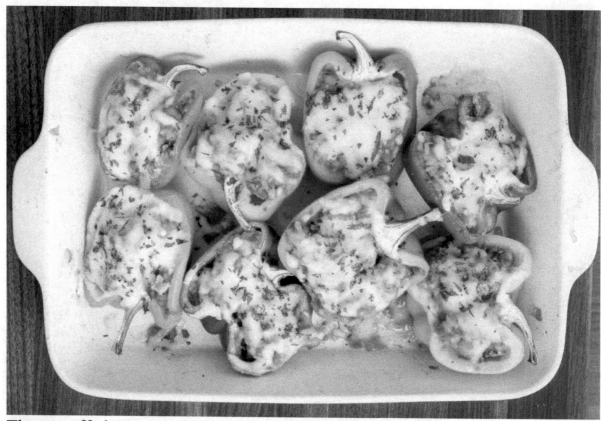

These stuffed peppers are easy to whip up and are extremely tasty.

**Serves:** 4

**Time:** 45 minutes

**Ingredients**

- 4 tbsp. shredded asiago cheese
- ¼ cup light ranch dressing
- 12-oz cooked, shredded chicken
- 1 tsp oil
- 1 red onion
- 4 large bell peppers of choice with tops cut and discarded, inside is hollowed out

**Directions**

1. Preheat oven to 375oF. On a baking dish, place peppers and bake for ten minutes to soften them.
2. Meanwhile, place a non-stick skillet on medium-high fire.

3. Sauté onion for 8 minutes, until soft.

4. In a bowl, mix well ranch dressing, sautéed onions, and shredded chicken.

5. Once peppers are done baking, evenly stuff with the chicken mixture and return to oven.

6. Bake for 30 minutes. When time is up, remove peppers, sprinkle cheese on top, and return to oven.

7. Broil for 3 minutes. 8. Serve and enjoy.

# Sheet Pan Healthy Chicken Parmesan

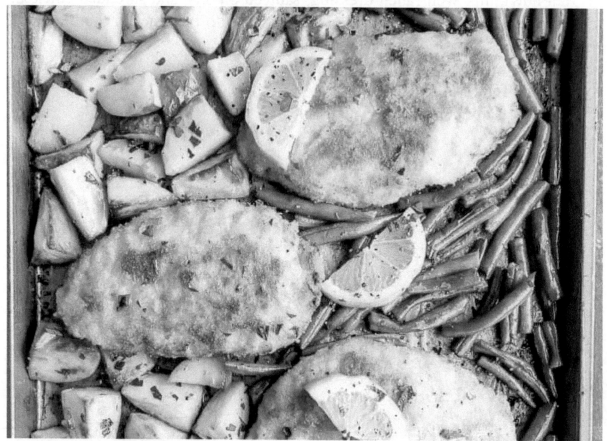

Here is a chicken parmesan recipe that is perfect if you are trying to avoid all the excess oil involved in deep frying.

**Serves:** 4

**Time:** 30 minutes

**Ingredients**

- ¼ cup panko bread crumbs
- ¼ cup grated parmesan cheese

- 1 tsp Italian seasoning
- Salt, 1 tsp., to taste
- Pepper, 1 tsp., to taste
- 1 tsp. garlic powder
- 1lb. chicken cutlets, skinless, boneless
- 1 egg, whisked
- 3 cups green beans
- 2 tsp. olive oil
- ½ cup marinara sauce, organic
- ½ cup fresh mozzarella cheese
- ¼ cup fresh basil, chopped

**Directions**

1. Set your oven to preheat to 4250F.

2. In a mixing bowl, combine the panko breadcrumbs, parmesan cheese, garlic powder, Italian seasoning, salt, and pepper.

3. Soak the chicken breasts into the egg and dredge onto the breadcrumb mixture.

4. Place on a baking sheet. Spray with cooking oil if desired. Toss the beans in olive oil and spread on the baking sheet with the chicken.

5. Cook for 15 minutes or until the chicken is cooked through.

6. Remove from the oven and pour the marinara sauce and mozzarella cheese. 7. Return to the oven and cook for 5 minutes or until the cheese melts. Top with fresh basil.

# Garlic Bacon and Cheese Stuffed Chicken Breasts

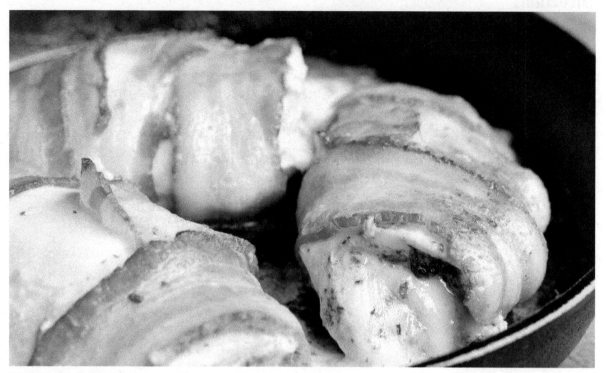

This chicken breast recipe produces a breast that is juicy, tender and extremely delicious.

**Serves:** 4

**Time:** 45 minutes

**Ingredients**

- 6 oz. chicken breasts, skinless
- 1 egg, beaten
- 2 tbsp. egg whites
- 2 ½ pounds bread crumbs
- 1 ½ tbsp. parmesan cheese, grated
- 2 tbsp. flour
- 1 ½ tsp. garlic powder
- 1 tsp Italian seasoning
- 4-ounce light cream cheese, softened
- 3 slices of bacon, cooked and crumbled
- 1 oz. light mozzarella cheese, shredded

**Directions**

1. Preheat the oven to 3750F.
2. Cut the chicken breasts open until it resembles a butterfly. Mix together the egg and egg whites in a bowl. Set aside.

3. In another bowl, combine the bread crumbs, parmesan cheese, flour, garlic powder, and Italian seasoning.

4. In another bowl, combine the cream cheese, and mozzarella cheese. Place a tbsp of the cheese mixture into the middle of the chicken breasts.

5. Place the flaps of meat over to close over the mixture. Secure with toothpicks.

6. Submerge the chicken in the egg mixture and dredge into the bread crumbs mixture. Place on a baking sheet.

7. Spray with cooking spray. Bake for 35 minutes until golden brown.

# Crispy Cheesy Baked Chicken Breasts

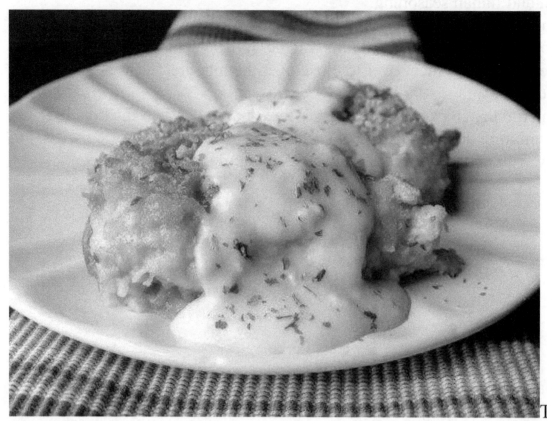

These chicken breasts are so crispy that you will believe they are deep fried.

**Serves:** 4

**Time:** 30 minutes

**Ingredients**

- Chicken Cutlets (1lb, skinless, boneless)
- Egg (1, whisked)

- Breadcrumbs (1/4 cup, panko)
- Garlic powder (1 tsp.)
- Italian seasoning (1 tsp.)
- Green beans (3 cups)
- Olive oil (2 tsp.)
- Marinara sauce (1/2 cup)
- Mozzarella cheese (1/2 cup, shredded)
- Basil (1/4 cup, chopped)

**Directions**

1. Set your oven to preheat to 425 degrees F then preparing a baking sheet by lightly greasing with cooking spray.

2. Add your Italian seasoning, garlic powder, salt, pepper, and breadcrumbs to a medium bowl.

3. Dredge your chicken into your egg then roll into your breadcrumb mixture.

4. Carefully place the chicken onto the baking sheet then lightly drizzle with olive oil.

5. Add your green beans to a large bowl, drizzle with olive oil and season to taste.

6. Toss to evenly coat. Add evenly around chicken pieces on the baking sheet.

7. Allow to cook until chicken has been fully cooked through (about 15 minutes).

8. When cooked, use your sauce and cheese to top your chicken pieces then return to the oven until your cheese is melted (about another 2 minutes).

9. Serve, and enjoy.

# Sticky Buffalo Chicken Tenders

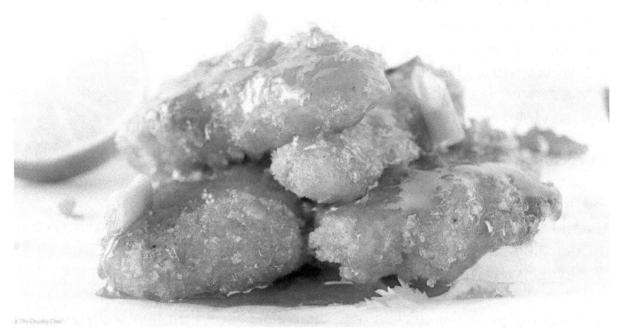

These chicken tenders be quickly become the star of any dinner party.

**Serves:** 6

**Time:** 30 mins.

**Ingredients**

- 1lb. skinless chicken breasts, pounded into ½" thickness
- ½ cup brown sugar
- 3 tablespoons water
- 3 eggs
- ¼ cup flour
- 1/3 cup red hot sauce
- 1 cup panko bread crumbs
- ½ teaspoon garlic powder

**Directions**

1. Preheat oven to 425 degrees F. Cut the chicken breasts into strips. Add chicken to a Ziploc bag and add the flour. Shake to coat.
2. Place the bread crumbs in a bowl. Place the egg in another bowl. Dip the floured meat into the eggs then into the breadcrumbs.
3. Add chicken to a baking sheet and spray with cooking oil on top. Bake in the oven for 20 minutes.

4. Meanwhile, make the sauce by mixing the remaining ingredients in a saucepan. 5. Toss your chicken tenders in your sauce and serve.

## Ham & Cheese Stuffed Chicken Breasts

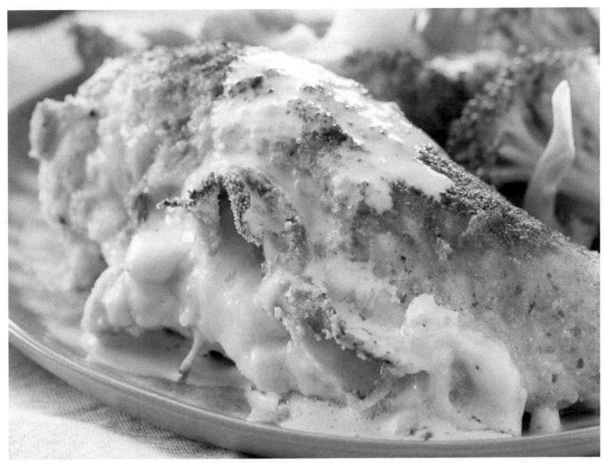

This delicious recipe combines breakfast and dinner together in one incredible dish.

**Serves:** 4

**Time:** 45 minutes

**Ingredients**

- 6 ounces skinless chicken breasts
- 1 egg, beaten
- 2 tbsp. egg whites
- 2 ½ pounds bread crumbs
- 1 ½ tbsp. parmesan cheese, grated
- 2 tbsp. flour
- 1 ½ tsp. garlic powder

- 1 tsp Italian seasoning
- 4-ounce light cream cheese, softened
- 3 slices of ham, cooked and crumbled
- 1-ounce light mozzarella cheese, shredded

## Directions

1. Preheat the oven to 3750F. Cut the chicken breasts open until it resembles a butterfly.
2. Mix together the egg and egg whites in a bowl. Set aside.
3. In another bowl, combine the bread crumbs, parmesan cheese, flour, garlic powder, and Italian seasoning.
4. In another bowl, combine the cream cheese, and mozzarella cheese. This will be the filling.
5. Place a tbsp of the cheese mixture into the middle of the chicken breasts.
6. Place the flaps of meat over to close over the mixture. Secure with toothpicks.
7. Submerge the chicken in the egg mixture and dredge into the bread crumbs mixture. Place on a baking sheet.
8. Spray with cooking spray.
9. Bake for 35 minutes until golden brown. 10. Serve and enjoy!

# Beef Roast

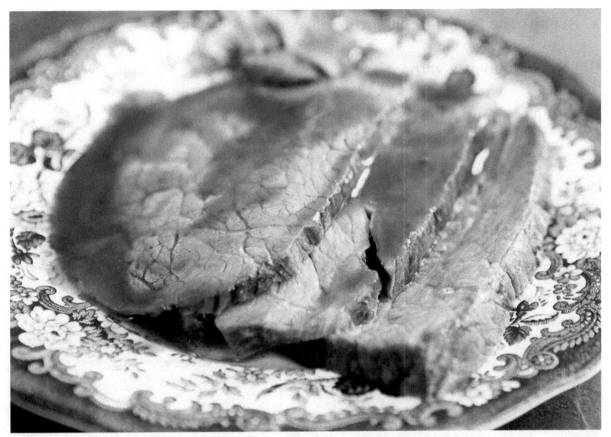

This delicious roast is tender, juicy and incredibly easy to make.

**Serves:** 8

**Time:** 1 hour 5 minutes

**Ingredients**

- 3 garlic bulbs
- 1 tablespoon lemon zest
- 2 tablespoons fresh thyme, chopped
- 3 teaspoons olive oil
- 3 ½ pounds boneless beef roast
- Salt and pepper, to taste

**Directions**

1. Preheat the oven to 350°F.
2. Line a roasting pan with parchment paper or foil. Mince 4 garlic cloves.
3. Mix minced garlic, lemon zest, 2 ½ teaspoons of olive oil, thyme, salt and pepper in a small bowl.
4. Rub the meat with the garlic mixture. Cut the top of the garlic bulbs.
5. Sprinkle the remaining oil on the cut surface of each bulb.

6. Put the prepared beef roast into the roasting pan along with garlic bulbs.

7. Place into the oven and bake for 60-65 minutes.

8. Remove the beef from the oven, cover with foil and let rest for at least 10 minutes before carving.

9. Serve with baked garlic cloves and spoon with some fat from the pan.

## Spicy Mexican Meatballs

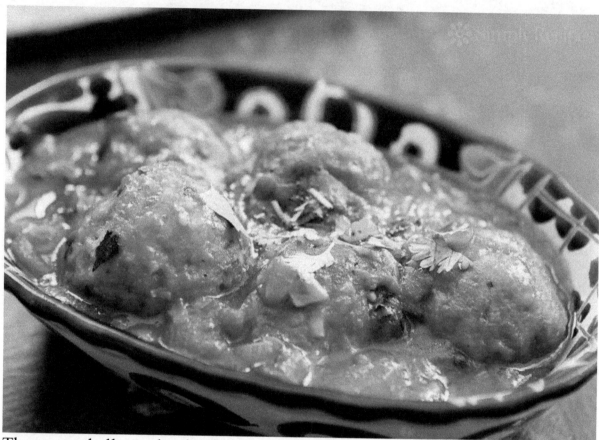

These meatballs are hardy, filling and overly yummy.

**Serves:** 4

**Time:** 45 minutes

**Ingredients**

- 1 lb. ground beef (92% lean)
- 4 oz. white onion, minced
- 4 oz. Monterey Jack cheese with spicy peppers
- 1 tablespoon butter
- 1 tablespoon ricotta cheese
- 3 cloves garlic

- 1 teaspoon chili powder
- 1 teaspoon ground cumin
- 1 teaspoon ground coriander
- 1 egg
- Sea salt and freshly ground pepper, to taste

## Directions
1. Preheat the oven to 350 F.
2. Heat butter in a frying pan, sauté onions until translucent. Set aside.
3. Shred and mince Monterey Jack cheese with spicy peppers. Set aside.
4. Whisk egg in a bowl and mix with ricotta cheese.
5. Add the spices, salt, and pepper and mix. Add onions and minced Monterey Jack cheese. Mix well.
6. Add beef and mix until all ingredients are combined. Form medium balls.
7. Place the meatballs on a cookie sheet and bake for about 20 minutes. 8. Serve and enjoy.

# Chocolate Berry Cheesecake

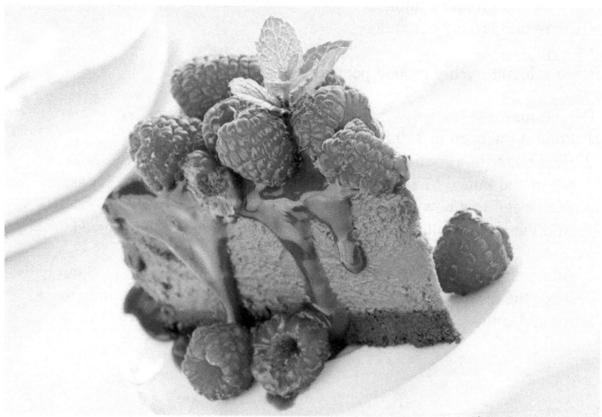

Finally, an easy dessert that can be pushed in the oven and ready in minutes.

**Serves:** 16

**Time:** 35 minutes

**Ingredients**

- 4 tablespoon butter, melted
- 1 ½ cup chocolate cookie, crumbed
- 3 packages low-fat cream cheese
- 2 tablespoon cornstarch
- 1 cup sugar
- 3 large eggs
- ½ cup plain Greek yogurt
- 1 tablespoon vanilla extract
- 4-ounce milk chocolate
- 4-ounce white chocolate
- 4-ounce bittersweet chocolate
- 1 cup sugared cranberries

**Directions**

1. Brush ramekins or a spring form pan with oil. Set aside.

2. Make the crust by combining butter with cookie crumbs. Press the dough at the bottom of the pan. Place in the freezer to set.

3. Beat the cream cheese with a mixer on low speed until smooth.

4. Add cornstarch and sugar and continue mixing until well combined.

5. Mix in eggs one at a time while continuing to beat. Scrape the sides of the bowl as needed.

6. Add the yogurt and vanilla and mix until well combined. Divide the batter in three bowls. Set aside.

7. Melt the milk chocolate in the microwave oven for 30 seconds twice until completely melted.

8. Whisk the chocolate into one of the bowls of the cheesecake batter. Do the same thing with the white and bittersweet chocolates.

9. Take the spring form pan out from the fridge. Pour the dark chocolate batter as the first layer, followed by the white chocolate and milk chocolate.

10. Put aluminum foil on top of the spring form pan. Pour water on the Instant Pot and place the steamer rack. Place the spring form pan and close the lid.

11. Cook on high for 10 minutes. Do a natural pressure release to open the lid.

12. Take the cheesecake out and refrigerate for 1 hour. 13. Serve with sugared cranberries.

## Cheesy Beef Casserole

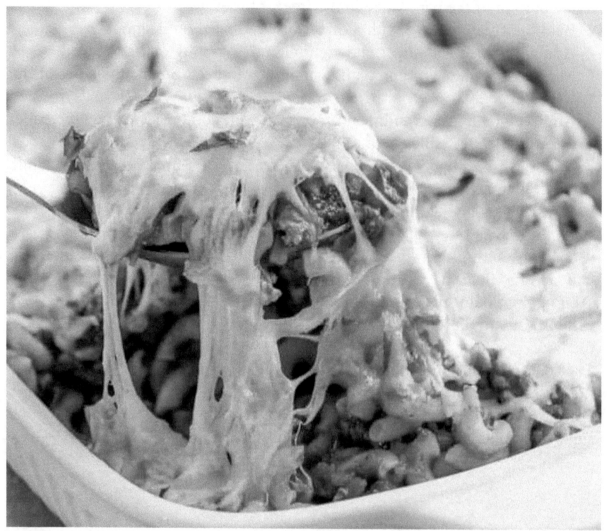

No Oven Cookbook would be complete without a delicious casserole. This recipe is easy to follow and extremely tasty.

**Serves:** 4

**Time:** 50 Minutes

**Ingredients:**

- 1 lb. lean ground beef
- 1 teaspoon vegetable oil
- 1 (15 ounce) can tomato sauce
- 10 ounces egg noodles, cooked
- 6 green onions, sliced
- 1 (15 ounce) can diced tomatoes
- ¾ teaspoon salt
- 1 cup cheddar cheese, grated
- ½ cup sour cream

- 1 cup low fat cottage cheese
- ½ green bell pepper, seeded and chopped
- 1 (3 ounce) package cream cheese, softened
- Salt, black pepper, to taste

**Instructions:**

1. Add oil into a large skillet and heat over medium heat for 2 minutes, add beef.
2. Cook for 5 minutes, add tomato sauce, tomatoes, and pepper, then season to taste. Simmer for 5 minutes.
3. Beat sour cream, cottage cheese, and cream cheese in a medium bowl with electric mixer.
4. Add onions and bell pepper then mix. Preheat the oven to 350 degrees F.
5. Coat a baking dish with cooking spray. Put one layer of half cheese mixture, second layer of half noodles and third layer of half meat mixture.
6. Repeat the layers then spread cheddar cheese on top.
7. Use foil to cover and allow to bake for about 20 minutes.
8. Remove the foil and bake for 10 more minutes. 9. Let rest for 5 minutes before serving. Enjoy!

# Conclusion

Congrats on making it all the way to the end. You did it! We hope you enjoyed all 30 delicious oven recipes that were featured in this Oven Cookbook and that it gave you a new appreciation for your oven.

So, what happens next?

Now for the big secret for mastering all 30 recipes, that's right I'm telling at the end, and that's because the secret is to keep on practicing. Nothing breathes perfection like practice. So, keep on cooking and enjoying these recipes over and over again. Then whenever you are ready for another spark of delicious inspiration grab another one of our books and let us continue our culinary journey together.

Remember to also drop us a review if you loved what you read and until we meet again, keep on cooking delicious food.

Lightning Source UK Ltd.
Milton Keynes UK
UKHW051525310521
384684UK00004B/701